About the author

From the Desk of Paul Webb

Paul Webb has been in the Health and Fitness business for over thirty years.

He has been actively serving his customers on-line since 1995.
Paul has several websites dedicated to Health and Fitness.

When Paul is not busy creating new products on health and fitness
he is spending time with his wife Linda helping raise his ten year old great-great-niece.

Some of Paul's sites are:
- Seniors Health Information
- Request Reviews
- Water Leak Repairs
- The Treadmill Report
- Saul To Paul

The Treadmill Repair Report alone, has helped thousands of people repair their treadmills.

Introduction

My name is Paul Webb; I am the owner of Electro Service Company.

I have been in the medical and fitness repair business for almost thirty years, and currently the supervisor of the Sterilizer repair shop at a major hospital in central Florida.

During the last thirty years I have repaired many brands of treadmills and fitness equipment. I decided to put this report together to help you diagnose and hopefully repair your treadmill at a fraction of the cost of having a technician come to your home or business.

Many of the problems with treadmills can be solved by a good preventive maintenance program or simple troubleshooting techniques. I have included many of these tips and techniques in this report.

I hope this report will save you the cost of a service call.

Please follow the directions in
the report and NEVER
Work on the treadmill with the
power on unless you feel
that you know what you are
doing!

It would be impossible to
cover every problem that can
happen with a treadmill. This
report will try to address
the most common problems.

***NEVER PERFORM ANY MAINTENANCE WITH THE POWER ON THE TREADMILL. ALWAYS UNPLUG ***

TREADMILL REPAIR

PREVENTIVE MAINTENANCE

The first and most important part of owning a treadmill or any piece of equipment is preventive maintenance. If you are not currently doing this then start today!

Items required for a good preventive maintenance program on your treadmill:

Vacuum cleaner
Screwdriver- Philip's and flat blade, sockets and Allen wrenches depending on your model.
Grease
Cleaning Rags

Now let's get started!

PLEASE ALWAYS
UNPLUG YOUR
TREADMILL
BEFORE DOING ANY
TYPE OF SERVICE

Remove the hood or motor
cover. There's probably
anywhere from 2 to 8
screws. Now vacuum the
dust from around the
motor and drive
mechanisms. What you
can't get to with the
vacuum use a small cloth
or brush. A clean motor
doesn't become clogged
and overheat.

After you have cleaned
around the motor, look for
any grease fittings, these
are usually found on
commercial grade units,
but your treadmill might
have some also.

For those of you who have never seen a grease fitting, they are about the size of a pencil eraser and have a hole in the end. They are usually found on bearings. If you don't have a grease gun you can buy a small gun and grease at your local auto parts store for less than $10.00.

If your unit is chain driven, clean the chain of excess dust, and apply a small amount of grease to the chain, also grease the drive chain and elevation chain as necessary.
Use white lithium grease if available.

Check all drive belts for wear, look for cuts and nicks, and replace as needed. Loosen the walking belt, most treadmills have either a bolt or screw on each side at the rear of the unit.

Loosen these, push the rear roller toward the walking deck until the belt is loose enough for you to look underneath.

Raise the belt and inspect the underside for wear. If it looks worn or burned you need to replace the belt.

Inspect the walking deck for wear, you will be able to tell if it's worn. If it has little ruts worn into it or bare spots it needs to be either flipped or replaced.

Many treadmills today have walking decks that can be flipped. If your deck is worn flip it, but it is recommended that when you flip the deck you replace the walking belt. If you need a new belt or deck we offer them here.
Treadmill Belts

Wipe the deck and
underside of the belt with
a soft cloth; depending on
your model of treadmill
you should lubricate
the walking deck at least
every 6 months. Some unit
use silicone spray or gel.
Others use wax. Check
your owner's manual for
what the manufacturer
recommends.

After you have cleaned the
belt and deck, and
lubricated the deck as
needed, center the belt on
the walking platform and
tighten the screws at the
end of the treadmill.

Turn each bolt the same
amount to keep the belt
centered. Tighten the belt
until it does not move
freely on the rollers.
Then with CAUTION
straddle the belt and start
the treadmill at low speed.

Wait for the belt to start moving then step on the belt. If it stops it is not tight enough. Step off the belt and tighten each side 1 turn then step on the belt again. Repeat as needed.

Once you can walk on the belt at low speed without it stopping or slipping increase the speed to 3 miles per hour. This should be a fast walk.

If your unit has side rails hold the rails and try to stop the belt with pressure.

IF ok then increase the speed to 5 MPH. Run on the treadmill, if you feel any slipping tighten the bolts another 1/2 turn each. Repeat if necessary.

If the belt is not centered, stand behind the treadmill and run the belt at full speed, if the belt is tracking to the left. Tighten the left bolt or screw 1/2 of a turn, and loosen the right bolt or screw 1/4 turn until the belt is centered.

IF the belt is tracking to the right, tighten the right side bolt or screw 1/2 turn and loosen the left bolt or screw 1/4 turn. Repeat as necessary, this should center the walking belt.

Always wipe the treadmill down after each use, perspiration is very corrosive.

If your treadmill inclines increase the elevation to maximum and vacuum underneath. If it doesn't incline pull it out and vacuum.

Most operating problems are easily seen, detected, and repaired. If the cause of a problem is not obvious, follow a logical process of checking each component in the system.

Repair of Your Treadmill

I t would be impossible for me to list every problem for every manufacturer's treadmill in this report, but here are some common problems:

Walking belt is not centered. See centering the belt procedure.

1. No power, check that the unit is plugged into a live outlet. **ALWAYS USE CAUTION** when dealing with electricity. Try another outlet if you need to. Remember K.I.S., and keep it simple.

If you know the outlet is live, unplug the unit and check the fuses.

Also check all connectors. You will need to lift the cover for this.

IF you have power but the motor does not turn you either have a bad power supply or the motor brushes are worn.

Contact the manufacturer for information. See the troubleshooting section.

If the motor is turning make sure the drive belt is not loose or broken. Tighten or replace as needed.

2. Walking belt moves, but there is a loud grinding noise.

Loosen the belt and see if the noise goes away, if it does you may have a bad front roller.

Sometimes you can spray the bearing in the roller with a lubricant like WD40 and this will solve the problem, but you may need to replace the roller.

If the noise does not go away then the motor bearings are probably bad and you will have to replace the motor or the motor bearings.

3. Elevation does not work, the treadmill will not go up or down or is stuck in the elevated mode.

Unplug the unit and check the elevation motor fuse, replace if necessary. Check the elevation system for broken chains or cables; make sure something hasn't gotten caught in the gears.

If your unit is equipped with limit switches for the up and down limits check them to be sure they are not engaged. These are usually little micro switches located around the elevation gears.

ALWAYS LOOK FOR LOOSE OR BROKEN WIRES FOR ANY PROBLEM YOU ARE HAVING.

4. You have power to the treadmill but the control panel does not work.

Check for loose wires or connections on the cables that go to the control panel.

If your treadmill has been in storage, or has not been used for any length of time it's possible that the connections on the cables have become corroded.

Unplug and clean, or
unplug and re-plug several
times to clean the
corrosion.

If your unit requires a key
or a magnet make sure it is
inserted correctly.
You may have a bad
control panel, and you will
need to replace it.

Check, for broken or loose
drive belts underneath the
cover.

5. The treadmill will run
for a short time then either
pops a fuse, or breaker or
just stops.

Probably the belt or deck,
or both, are worn and need
to be replaced.

Check the belt tension it
might be too tight, and is
causing the motor to
overheat and stop. Try
lubricating the deck first.

If this does not help
then you will need to
replace the worn parts.
You should also inspect
the belt and deck for wear.

How to Measure Your Treadmill Belt for Replacement

If your treadmill is not a
major brand and it needs a
new belt you may have to
special order a belt.
Following are instruction
for making sure you get a
good measurement.

Next to the motor the
treadmill belt is the most
important part of the
treadmill. If it becomes
frayed or starts to turn up
on the sides then it
is time to replace the belt.

The treadmill belt will
also split at the seam. You
should check the belt on a
regular basis.

This will ensure it is safe. If the belt wears thin it can ruin the deck, then you have the double expense of replacing the belt and deck.

We sell replacement treadmill belts, and take special orders. But you must have the correct measurement so your belt will fit. Following are the directions to measure your belt.

To measure your treadmill belt for replacement do the following:

1. Place a mark on the edge of the belt, then using a string or tape measure goes completely around the belt to get the circumference. This needs to be as close as you can get it.

2. Measure the width of the belt.

Example 102" X 15"

If your belt is so bad that you know it has to be replaced then could cut it off and measure the entire length and width of the belt. If it is a very old belt please allow for stretching.

You can also set the rear roller about halfway of the adjusting screws then measure around the front and rear rollers for an accurate measurement.
To order belts use the link below.

http://treadmills.cc/store/

How to Replace Your Treadmill Belt

Is your treadmill belt worn, torn, or curling up on the edges? Does your treadmill slow down after you step on the belt and begin your workout?

If this is the case then it may be time to replace the belt.

Here are some things to check before replacing your belt.

1. You need to make sure the deck of the treadmill is in good shape. If it looks good then it may only need to be waxed or lubricated.

2. If the deck shows obvious signs of wear, or has grooves worn into it then you may need to

replace the belt and the deck.

3. If the deck looks good, and the belt is worn or starting to turn up on the edges then it is time to replace the belt. Here are the instructions for doing that. Most treadmills are basically the same so this is a generic set of instructions. If you have an owner manual please follow the manufacturer's instructions.

To begin the belt replacement, unplug the POWER Cord and remove the motor cover or hood. Then locate the screws or bolts that are used to adjust the belt tension. They are normally on either side at the rear of the treadmill. Loosen both sides and push the rear roller toward the deck.

Now loosen and remove
the front roller. If your
treadmill inclines,
turn on the power and
raise the treadmill a few
degrees so the roller can
be removed. After the
front roller is removed,
remove the rear roller.
Now you are ready to
remove the belt.

I know it would be easier
to just cut the old belt off,
but if you take it off
in one piece then you will
remember how to put the
new one on.

Along the sides of the
treadmill you will find
bolts or screws that hold
the deck in place. Remove
these and lift the deck and
old belt out together.
Now is the time to wax or
lubricate the deck.

Look at the old belt and the new belt. There will probably be a visible seam on the belt. Normally the belt should be installed so that the seam goes downward from left to right, much like a backward slash.

Some belt manufacturers will mark the belt on the inside with an arrow pointing in the direction the belt should travel.

Slide the belt over the deck in the proper alignment and lay the belt and deck together back onto the treadmill. Start all of the screws or bolts before tightening them securely. Decks tend to get warped after a while.

Pull the belt to the rear of the treadmill and slide the rear roller through it. Start the adjusting screws in the roller just enough so they do not fall out.

Now slide the front roller inside the belt and replace the drive motor belt over the drive gear. Do this before you tighten the roller.

After you get the front roller tight, then tighten the deck bolts and the rear roller with the adjusting screws. Tighten each side equally until the belt feels snug on the deck.

Now turn the treadmill on. If the belt starts moving, carefully step on the treadmill while holding the side rails.

If the belt stops then you need to adjust more. Step off the treadmill, and tighten each screw one full turn and step on the belt again. Repeat this process until the belt does not stop.

Now increase the speed to a fast walk, hold the handrails and apply downward pressure as you walk on the treadmill.

If the belt stops or hesitates then adjust some more. Now increase the speed to a jog, probably around 5 m.p.h. Once again if you feel hesitation in the belt when your foot hits it, adjust it some more. Continue these processes until you are satisfied that the belt is not slipping.

PLEASE be careful, if you do not think you can do this then pay someone to do it for you.

Please follow these directions for safe and efficient use of your treadmill for you and your family.

If you have recently moved the treadmill or have changed the power outlet where it is connected, then make sure that the outlet is not the problem.

Check the breakers in your electrical panel, and the power cord for cuts, or loose plugs.

1. The treadmill will not run at all, or runs for a few minutes then shuts off. The problem could be A,B,C,D, or E.

A. Check the electrical plug for a loose connection, and repair if needed.

B. The motor brushes may be bad. Unplug the unit and remove the motor cover.

C. If your motor has brushes, remove and inspect the brushes for wear. They should be worn evenly. If not then one of them is not making good contact.

While you have both brushes out of the motor use a can of air or blow through the brush holders really hard. You will probably see carbon come out of the motor.

If you need new brushes you can probably match them up at a local small motor repair shop, or call the manufacturer.

D. The speed sensor could be dirty or out of adjustment. While you have the motor cover off, clean around the motor with the vacuum. If your unit has a speed sensor it will be located near the flywheel of the motor.

Clean the sensor and make sure it almost touches the flywheel. Also check for loose connections. Sometimes you can cure a problem by simply unplugging, then reconnecting a connector.

If your unit elevates then do the same thing for the elevation sensor, and the upper and lower limit switches.

E. This could be because the deck or belt or possibly both are worn and need to be replaced. Loosen the rear roller and push it toward the deck.

F. This should give you enough space to look underneath the belt and inspect it and the deck.

If the belt is "burned", it will look black and slick.

If the deck is worn you may see grooves in the top of the deck. Or you will see that the lubrication is worn off the deck.

If your deck is a "slick deck", they are normally black, and the wax is white.

If the wax is gone you will probably see some at the front of the deck and some at the rear, but none in the middle. You can try waxing or lubricating the deck.

If your unit uses a key or magnet to operate, try moving it around and see if the treadmill will start.

If you have lost the key, some of my customers have told me that they used an old credit card folded in half to fit into the slot. All the key does is close a micro switch, so anything that will close the switch will work.

2. Loud noise coming from the rollers or drive belt.

A. If the loud squeal is coming from under the hood of the treadmill then it could be the drive belt or the front roller. Remove the hood and start the treadmill, you should be able to tell where the noise is coming from.

If it is from the drive belt, perhaps it is worn and needs to be replaced or the tension is not right. The procedure for adjusting the drive belt is below.

B. If the front or rear roller is squealing, you may be able to stop it by spraying the end of the roller with a silicone lubricant.

If that doesn't work, and the bearings can be replaced, then replace them. It's not that hard. The bearing is usually held in by a locking ring.

Remove the locking ring from each end and find something that will slide inside the roller to knock the bearings out. You can take the old bearing to your local gear and wheel shop and match them up. They may even remove the old ones and re-install the new ones for you.

C. If the motor bearings are squealing then take the motor out and take it to a shop to have the bearings replaced.

Control Panel Does Not Work

Take the cover off and look for fuses that go to the control panel.

Perhaps the connections
are corroded, unplug all
connectors and re-plug
them a few times, also
check for broken or
loose connections, and
broken or loose wires. Pay
special attention to the
ones that go up to the
control panel.

Some control panels are
battery operated, check to
make sure you don't have
bad batteries.

How to Adjust the Motor Drive Belt

The motor drive belt needs to be adjusted from time to time, especially if you have adjusted the walking belt. If your drive belt is loose it will slip on the pulley of the front roller and can cause the walking belt to slip or skip.

If it is too tight it will draw too much current and could damage the motor or the front roller. However too tight is better than too loose.

To check for proper tension on the drive belt try the procedure I outlined for stopping the belt while it is moving about 3mph. The cover must be off so you can watch the drive belt.

While walking about 3mph apply pressure on the walking belt. If the drive belt stops or slips then it needs to be tightened.

If your unit has a belt tensioning adjustment bolt then tighten it. There may be a locknut on this bolt. Loosen the locking nut and tighten the tension bolt. You will need to loosen the motor mount bolts before doing this.

If you do not have a motor tension bolt, you will have to loosen the motor mounts. This will require two people. After the bolts are loose one person will need to apply pressure to the motor to tighten the drive belt while the other person tightens the bolts.

Repeat the testing process until the drive belt no longer slips.

If you have problems let
me know.

How To Replace The Motor Drive Belt

First thing you need to
do is loosen the tension
on the walking belt,
then push the rear roller
toward the deck.

Now loosen and remove
the bolts holding the
front roller. You may
only have to remove the
one on the drive pulley
side.

Slip the new belt over
the drive pulley and the
roller pulley and re-
install the front roller.

If needed loosen the
motor mounts just
enough to allow you to
slip the belt over the
drive pulley.

If you have to loosen
the drive motor to get
the new belt over the
pulley, then loosen the
motor mounts, and push
the motor towards
the treadmill deck.

Once you have it on
then pull the drive motor
back to tighten the belt.

You may need a second
person the hold tension
on the motor while you
tighten the mounting
bolts.

Once you have the belt
installed then adjust the
walking belt tension
using the instructions
above for adjusting the
belt tension.

Please feel free to contact me with your specific problem, and I may be able to help you more.

We offer walking belts for any treadmill: http://treadmills.cc/store/

If you do not see your model listed then we can special order the belt. We will need the exact measurements of your belt. Use the directions in this report for measuring.

Please Read:

If you feel The Treadmill Report has helped you solve your treadmill problem, then I would like to hear from you.

*** NEVER PERFORM ANY MAINTENANCE WITH THE POWER ON THE TREADMILL. ALWAYS UNPLUG ***

TESTIMONIALS

Thank you Paul for your info. The problem was right in my face. If I didn't read your report I would have lost a lot of money. Thank you.

Nikki

Thanks Paul! I fixed my treadmill! Before I fixed it, the motor ran and the walking belt moved, but as soon as you stepped on it, the walking belt stopped. It had a loose motor belt - once I tightened it, it worked normally. Thanks for your advice!

Tom

A great big thank you for the report. I think I solved my problem. The motor makes a humming noise and the screens are all blank.

The power went off for
just second while I was on
the treadmill and it quit
running. But I think your
report helped. Appreciate
your consideration.

Arnold

Paul- Thanks for the
report. Yes, your report
would have helped but
I called a treadmill repair
service and he found and
repaired the problem
in 15 minutes for his
minimum charge of
$120.00!

I had a speed sensor
problem with my Model
One Treadmill. You
addressed this problem in
your Troubleshooting Tips
section 1.C. Wished I had
emailed you earlier for
your report and saved
some money!

Bill

PLEASE ALWAYS
UNPLUG YOUR
TREADMILL BEFORE
DOING
ANY TYPE OF
SERVICE

Sincerely,
Paul Webb
http://treadmills.cc
admin@treadmills.cc

List of Manufacturers

Bodyguard 418-228-8934
Bodymaster 800-325-8964
Bollinger 800-527-1166
Challenger 800-374-4121
Cybex 800-677-6544
Landice 800-526-3423
Lifefitness 800-351-3737
Marquette 800-558-5102
Pacer 800-651-6119
Paramount 213-721-2121
Precor 800-786-8404
x200
Preference 800-776-7641
Proform 800-999-3756
Quinton 800-426-0337
Spirit 800-258-8511
Stairmaster 800-635-2936

Tectrix 800-767-8082

Trackmaster 800-396-1570

Trotter 800-677-6544 x6163

Tunturi 800-736-7616

Unisen 800-503-1221(also known as Startrac)

Universal 800-553-7901

Weslo 800-999-3756

RBTL1198 Reebok ACD1
Voltage Diagram

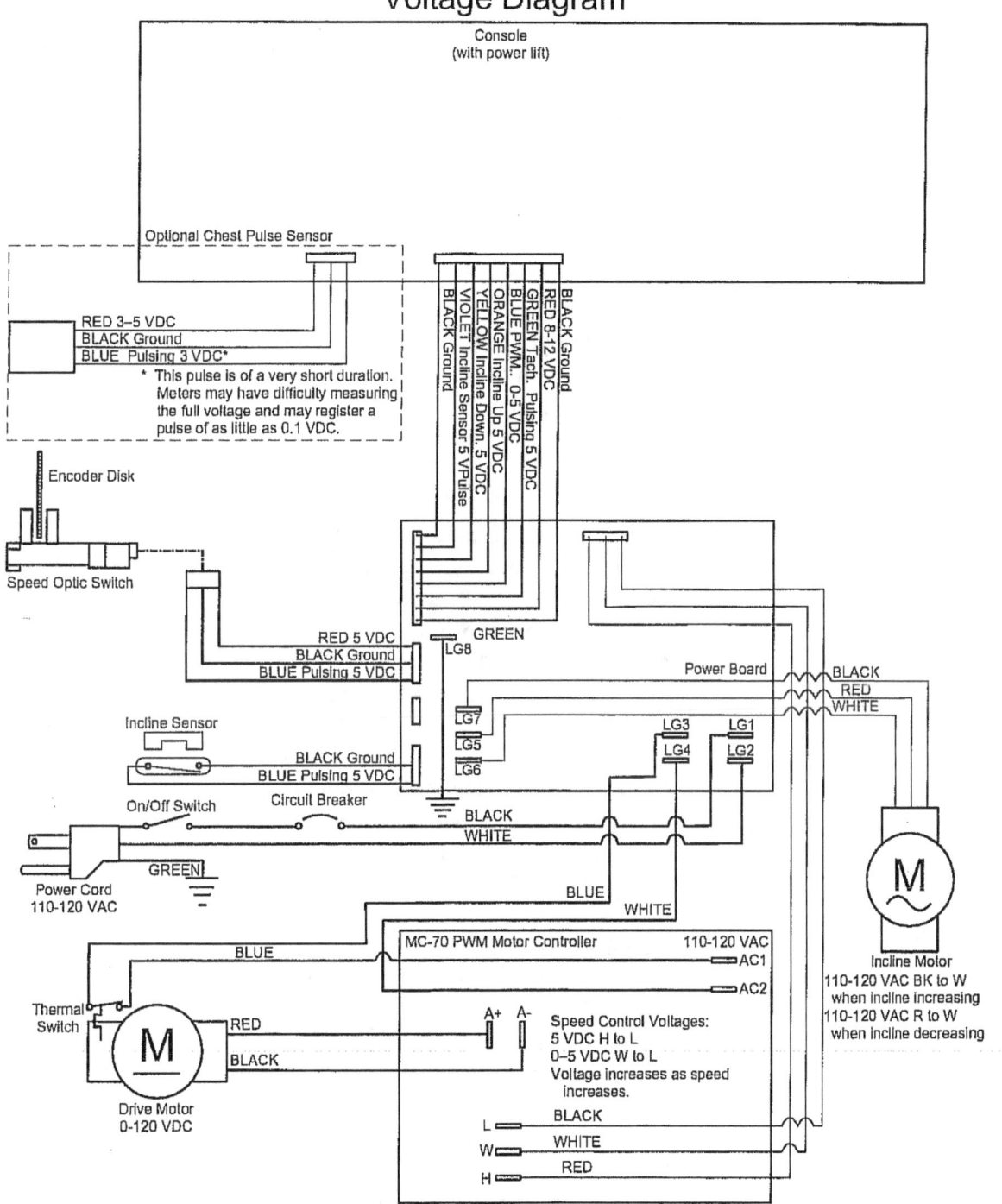

Part #: 149583 10/98 Drawing #: H03415-A

From: Joe
To: Paul

Dear Paul,

I need to replace my motor drive
belt as your ad states is in this
book.
"How to adjust, and replace the
motor drive belt."

Joe,

First thing you need to do is loosen
the tension on the walking belt,
then push the rear roller toward the
deck.

Now loosen and remove the bolts
holding the front roller. You may
only have to remove the one on the
drive pulley side. Slip the new belt
over the drive pulley and the roller
pulley and re-install the front roller.

If needed loosen the motor mounts
just enough to allow you to slip the
belt over the drive pulley.

If you have to loosen the drive
motor to get the new belt over the
pulley, then loosen the motor
mounts, and push the motor
towards the treadmill deck.

Once you have it on then pull the
drive motor back to tighten the belt.
You may need a second person the
hold tension on the motor while
you tighten the mounting bolts.

Once you have the belt installed then adjust the walking belt tension using the instructions in the treadmill report.

Paul

Hello,

I have a Proform treadmill, and I've tried tightening the belt but it continues to slip when I get on the treadmill. The belt runs fine until I get on the treadmill and then it starts slipping. What other issues could I be having with it?

Thanks,
James

James,

Remove the cover and make sure the motor drive belt is not slipping, it could be loose therefore causing the walking belt to stall. There is a procedure in the report for tightening the drive belt.

Have you tried the test in the report where you tighten the belt at 3 mph, then 5mph. If not do that.

Get on the treadmill and increase the speed to 3mph, and apply hard pressure to try and stall the belt. Watch the drive belt for slippage while doing this. If the walking belt stalls and the drive belt does not slip.

Then tighten the belt until you can't make it slip at 3.
Then increase to 5mph and do the same thing.

If the motor drive belt is not loose and you run out of adjustment for the walking belt then the belt may be stretched.

The only thing you can do then is replace the belt.

Let me know

Paul

From: Florante
To: Paul

Dear Mr. Webb,

Thank you for providing me with the Report. Nevertheless, I still have my problem unresolved since it involves replacing the motor drive belt.

I own a Trimline 7150 treadmill, which has been discontinued and subsequently bought and absorbed by Nautilus. I bought the drive belt but I don't know how to install it. I don't know which part to remove first.

I have the exploded view of the parts as provided when I initially bought it but it does not show or instruct which part to remove first to free up the worn out belt. I'm afraid that if I just go ahead and unscrewing the nearest bolt I might end up with a heap of metal junk. I need a "how-to" step-by-step instruction manual on how to replace the motor drive belt.

Help!!

Florante,

Here are the steps:

1. Loosen the rear roller bolts, but do not remove them, and push the roller toward the deck, or front of the treadmill.

2. Remove the hood or motor cover, and remove the bolts that hold the front roller in place.

3. Drop the front roller enough to slide the old belt off, then replace the new motor drive belt over the roller pulley and the motor pulley.

4. Replace the front roller and secure. You may have to loosen the motor mounts a liitle, but put them back where they were after the belt is installed.

5. Tighten the rear roller bolts, use the procedures in the treadmill report for tightening the belt so it does not slip.

Thanks,

Paul

Hi,

Yes, I did find your info. Helpful......My treadmill powers up and even reclines up and down, but the belt does not move and I did not see a resolution for that on your site, although I know that it is impossible to have everything listed. Do you have some idea as to what could be wrong?

Thanks for your help!

Kim

Hello Kim,

A few thing to check.
1. Does the front roller turn?

2. If not then remove the cover and make sure the drive belt from the motor to the front roller is not broken, loose or has slipped off.

3. UNPLUG THE TREADMILL--- If the drive belt is ok, check the fuses, and connections to the motor, and the motor brushes.

4. If your unit has a speed sensor (it will be located on or near the flywheel of the motor) make sure that it is not loose or dis-connected. It should be almost touching the flywheel.

5. If your unit requires a magnet or key, make sure it is making a good connection.

Paul

----- Original Message -----
From: Walter
To: Paul
Subject: treadmill for Sears
Lifestyler 5.0

Dear Sir...
 I've just ordered your product for the treadmill report, but still having a problem. I have a Sears Lifestyler 5.0 that has a bad treadmill belt that needs replaced. I already have the replacement belt and have loosened the rear bolts that keep the belt tight, but I can't find a bolt or screw that will allow me to take the old walking belt off and put the new one on. Any help would be greatly appreciated.
Thanks!!

Walter

Walter,

After you loosen the rear roller, push it forward, then loosen and remove the front roller. If the treadmill inclines this will easier.

After you remove the front roller,
there should be cover plates where
the rear roller bolts go, remove the
rear bolts, then the cover plates and
remove the rear roller.

Your treadmill may have side
covers, that hide the deck screws,
remove these covers and you
will find the bolts that hold the
deck to the frame. Or possibly the
deck slides out from the rear.
Remove the deck and belt together.

Remove the deck and belt, install
the new belt over the deck and
replace both back into the machine.
Slide the rear roller through the belt
and put it in place then push it up
against the deck.

Now slide the front roller through
the belt and put the drive belt from
the motor back on the front roller
then secure the roller to the
treadmill frame.

Now put the rear roller cover
plates, and the bolts into the rear
roller and start tightening the belt.

Follow the belt replacement
procedures in The Treadmill Report
to adjust the belt.

Use CAUTION when testing the
belt for proper tightness.

Paul

----- Original Message -----
From: Michel
To: Paul

The problem I have is the treadmill overheating and cutting out.

If you have any specific ideas on this do let me know.

M.

Michael,

Have you checked the deck for wear, and the underside of the belt for wear. It sounds like your belt is probably dragging on the deck instead of slipping over it, this cause the motor to work to hard, and eventually overheat.

Loosen the belt enough to look underneath, inspect the deck for wear. If you see grooves or the finish is worn off, then it needs to be waxed or flipped. If it is a black deck check the other side and see if it has wax on it. If so you can flip the deck.

If you can flip the deck you probably need to replace the belt. Check the underside of the belt for wear while you have it loose.

Read this article:

Is your treadmill belt worn, torn or curling up on the edges? Does your treadmill slow down after you step on the belt and begin your workout?

If this is the case then it may be time to replace the belt.

Here are some things to check before replacing your belt.

1. You need to make sure the deck of the treadmill is in good shape. If it looks good then it may only need to be waxed or lubricated.

2. If the deck shows obvious signs of wear, or has grooves worn into it then you may need to replace the belt and the deck.

3. If the deck looks good, and the belt is worn or starting to turn up on the edges then it is time to replace the belt. Here are the instructions for doing that.
Most treadmills are basically the same so this is a generic set of instructions. If you have an owners manual please follow the manufacturers instructions.

To begin the belt replacement unplug the POWER Cord and remove the motor cover or hood.

Then locate the screws or bolts that are used to adjust the belt tension. They are normally on either side at the rear of the treadmill. Loosen both sides and push the rear roller toward the deck.

Now loosen and remove the front roller. If your treadmill inclines, turn on the power and raise the treadmill a few degrees so the roller can be removed. After the front roller is removed, remove the rear roller. Now you are ready to remove the belt.

I know it would be easier to just cut the old belt off, but if you take it off in one piece then you will remember how to put the new one on. Along the sides of the treadmill you will find bolts or screws that hold the deck in place. Remove these and lift the deck and old belt out together. Now is the time to wax or lubricate the deck.

Look at the old belt and the new belt. There will probably be a visible seam on the belt. Normally the belt should be installed so that the seam goes downward from left to right, much like a backward slash. Some belt manufacturers will mark the belt on the inside with an arrow pointing in the direction the belt should travel.

Slide the belt over the deck in the proper alignment, and lay the belt and deck together back onto the treadmill. Start all of the screws or bolts before tightening them securely.

Decks tend to get warped after a while so you may need to push or pull a little to get the screws started. I have found that it is a good idea to install the rollers before securely fastening the deck to the frame.

Pull the belt to the rear of the treadmill and slide the rear roller through it. Start the adjusting screws in the roller just enough so they do not fall out. Now slide the front roller inside the belt and replace the drive motor belt over the drive gear. Do this before you tighten the roller.

After you get the front roller tight, then tighten the rear roller with the adjusting screws. Tighten each side equally until the belt feels snug on the deck.

Now turn the treadmill on. If the belt starts moving, carefully step on the treadmill while holding the side rails. If the belt stops then you need to adjust more. Step off the treadmill, and tighten each screw one full turn and step on the belt again. Repeat this process until the belt does not stop.

Now increase the speed to a fast walk, hold the handrails and apply downward pressure as you walk on the treadmill. If the belt stops or hesitates then adjust some more. Now increase the speed to a jog, probably around five mph. Once again if you feel hesitation in the belt when your foot hits it, adjust it some more. Continue this process until you are satisfied that the belt is not slipping.

PLEASE be careful, if you do not think you can do this then pay someone to do it for you.

Please follow these directions for safe and efficient use of your treadmill for you and your family.

If you need a belt I do have belts for most treadmills available at the website.

I hope this helps.

Thanks
Paul

----- Original Message -----
From: Cho
To: Paul

Dear Paul,

Thank you very much for the treadmill report. This is a great help for people like me with little knowledge about treadmill. Let me take this opportunity to tell you the exact problem of my treadmill.

It seems that it its running 2.6 kph SLOWER than what is displayed by the digital controller. when the error is sensed by the controller, treadmill stops. Do you think the defect is contributed by the motor itself?

I have spent money paying the technician and yet problem is still not known. What can you advise? Thank you and I hope I can hear from you.

Regards,
Cho

Cho,

  You could have a dirty speed sensor, or the deck and belt could be worn, which would slow the belt down. How do you know the belt is actually running slower than the display reads? Did the technician measure the speed with a tachometer?

I don't know what kind of treadmill you have, but some models have a calibration program that will actually calibrate the speed sensor to the motor speed.

But I would clean the sensor and motor area. You might want to check and see if the sensor is positioned correctly, perhaps it has moved from the vibration of the treadmill.

If you feel safe doing this, start the treadmill at 1 mph or kph, then

loosen the sensor and, while the
belt is running, move the sensor
around to see if the indicated speed
increases, or decreases. If so then
place it where it reads 1kph.

I hope this helps.

Thanks
Paul

----- Original Message -----
From: Moe
To: admin@treadmills.cc

Thank you for your report on fixing
treadmills. I can't find any
troubleshooting tips that apply
to our situation so I thought I would
email you and see if you could
help. I tried calling NordicTrack
for help but that was in vain.

Our NordicTrack is 2 years old.
Unfortunately nowhere in the
manual does it give maintenance
tips. When I asked why not they
replied they just decided not to
include it.

Our walking deck squeaks badly.
We have used the lube under the
walking belt but it didn't help.
It is not the front roller or the back
roller. It is coming from under the
deck, perhaps the liner underneath.
Is there anything we can do to get
rid of this annoying squeak?

Hello,

I'm not sure how your deck is mounted to the frame, but on the old trackmaster it was mounted with 6 rubber bumpers. Sometimes one of these would crack in half, and would start squeaking. It was hard to find, I had to raise the treadmill and loosen them to find the bad one.

Perhaps this is your problem also. if not then have someone walk on the treadmill while you listen as close as possible all the way around the edge where the deck meets the frame.

You can probably isolate it down to where the squeak is coming from, then cut a small piece of door insulation,(the stuff you buy at home depot to put around your door frame to keep the wind out) . Place this between the deck and the frame to stop the squeak.

Also raise the treadmill if possible, and crawl underneath and inspect with a flashlight, where the deck and frame are connected. This is one of those annoying problems you just have to look for until you find it. Wish I could be more help, but if you do the things above you will probably find the squeak.

One more thing; Remove the cover and have someone run on the treadmill while you watch the belt that goes from the motor to the front roller. If it "jumps" every their foot hits the deck then that might also be your squeak. Tighten the drive belt or apply belt dressing.

Thanks, Paul

----- Original Message -----
From: Jeff
To: admin@treadmills.cc

Paul,

Thank you for the response. I went through your process and still haven't found the problem.

Here's the deal. I have a Life Fitness TR3500 treadmill. I plug it in and try to start it up and nothing happens. I get a 'Start Error' message on the display.

When this first occurred, I heard a sound similar to a fuse blow and smelled something burning. Whether this was a fuse, the control board, transformer, motor, or other-I do not know. I can pull the belt by hand and the motor turns, would a burnt-out motor be able to do that?

Any guidance here would be greatly appreciated.

Thank you, Jeff

Hello Jeff,

To answer your question, it's more
likely that you have a bad start cap
for the motor.They will usually pop
if the short out. Inspect all of the pc
boards and associated electronics
for evidence of burning. Sometimes
I will unplug the treadmill and get
as close to the board as possible
and sniff the components. If one
has blown you will smell it.

If your motor has a start cap it will
be mounted on the motor or in the
near vicinity of the motor.
These can be replaced, go to a local
electronic barn or someplace that
sells surplus electronic parts and
find a replacement capacitor. A
small motor repair shop could
probably help you. Take the cap
with you.

Paul
admin@treadmills.cc

----- Original Message -----
From: Joshua
To: Paul

My treadmill is slipping as I try to
run on it.
I have replaced the rear belt
adjusters.

The belt is self greased on the running board I have the front roller to replace it haven't yet.
 I have adjusted the tension many many, many, many, many times.I am at the end of my rope give me some tips.

Thanks,
Joshua

Joshua,

It sounds like the belt is stretched and probably needs to be replaced. If you have adjusted it many times and the belt tension screws are maxed out, that is a pretty good indicator that it is stretched.

How old is the treadmill and have you ever replaced the belt?

I do offer belts if you need a new one.
http://treadmills.cc/store/

Thanks,

Paul

www.ingramcontent.com/pod-product-compliance
Lightning Source LLC
Chambersburg PA
CBHW081858280526
45789CB00007B/2756